Getting People Involved in Life and Activities

Effective Motivating Techniques

Getting People Involved in Life and Activities

Effective Motivating Techniques

by

Jeanne Adams, M.S., C.T.R.S., A.C.C.

Venture Publishing, Inc.
State College, Pennsylvania

Copyright © 1995

Venture Publishing, Inc.
1999 Cato Avenue
State College, PA 16801
(814) 234-4561 FAX (814) 234-1651

No part of the material protected by this copyright notice may be reproduced or utilized in any form or by any means, electronic or mechanical, including photocopying, recording, or by any information storage and retrieval system, without written permission from the copyright owner.

Trademarks: All brand names and product names used in this book are trademarks, registered trademarks or trade names of their respective holders.

Production Manager: Richard Yocum
Design, Layout, and Graphics: Diane K. Bierly
Manuscript Editing: Diane K. Bierly
Additional Editing: Katherine Young and Richard Yocum
Cover Art and Design: Sandra Sikorski, Sikorski Design 1995

Library of Congress Catalogue Card Number 95-61706
ISBN 0-910251-78-9

To John and Loretta Adams

Who by their example taught each of their ten children the value of becoming positively involved in life.

Table of Contents

Section I

Chapter 1 Why Do They *Just Sit There*? 3
A brief summation of some of the main reasons for lack of motivation for activity involvement.

Chapter 2 What Do They Really Need From *Me*? 7
Descriptions of the major needs of people receiving planned activity services.

Chapter 3 Natural Motivators 11
A listing of no-cost, life-enriching experiences that naturally motivate people for further involvement.

Section II

Chapter 4 Practical Motivators 17
This chapter lists readily usable techniques for getting and keeping people involved in activity programs.

Chapter 5 Their Greatest Motivation 49
The importance of being yourself and the importance of relationships: How these affect the individual and the group.

Appendix: Practical Exercises 51

References and Additional Reading 55

Section I

Chapter 1

Why Do They *Just Sit There*?

Motivation, especially motivation for involvement in life activities, is the biggest challenge and most frustrating task facing therapeutic recreation staff no matter whom they are serving. The ability to motivate someone toward increasing his or her quality of life is what distinguishes the truly effective therapeutic recreation leader from the average worker. (Please note: Although the term "therapeutic recreation" is used throughout, my comments and ideas are directed at all who provide planned activity programming.)

All life is activity. As human beings, we spend our entire lives moving in and through our changing environments with varying energy levels, goals, and motivations connected with activity. When we feel good about ourselves and in control of our personal world, we are able to move with direction and purpose. We are alive and open to new experiences. There is an awareness of genuine self-worth and our actions and decisions are easily initiated. We feel a sense of community while maintaining a strong value base that keeps a perspective on life. Our thoughts and senses are generally tuned to the positive, and our self-messages are encouraging. We know who we are, and we live what we believe. We are in balance.

The motivation which goes with this sense of balance is considered to be "a psychobiological condition in which the individual is oriented towards, and tries to achieve, some kind of fulfillment" (Bromley, 1990). When we are in this state of active fulfillment, when we feel good about ourselves, we are motivated to move towards involvement in life and activity.

Within a healthy individual there is a feeling of independence as well as interdependence. It is an awareness that one has value and has something to offer others. The need to feel that one's contribution to society is recognized and fulfilled. A true personal identity coexists with a sense of belonging (Frye and Peters, 1972).

One of the most vital things that you as a therapeutic recreation leader, have to offer a person can best be described by an old Native American saying: "Give me a fish and I eat for a day. Teach me to fish and I eat for a lifetime." Give me something and I have it for a moment; help me to discover it myself and I carry it with me always.

What seems to be characteristic of a well-intentioned, yet *ineffective* therapeutic recreation leader, is behavior that, for the most part, "does for" or "gives to" another. Although this type of helping behavior might feel right to the "giver" and may even be more expedient at times, it has tremendous potential for creating dependency and a sense of learned helplessness. In effect, the other person becomes the "model patient," no matter what term we might use in referring to him or her. Along with this "patient" identification goes a sense of having been reduced in stature, ability, and responsibility. Often the resident develops a victim mentality, leading to further passivity and dependence on others. "Activity—action—is the vital component of all change. Without change, recovery (e.g., rehabilitation, restitution) is illusory. Without activity and change, which is life itself, there is no growth" (Erikson, 1976).

Perhaps the number one goal of a therapeutic recreation leader is to increase the quality of life for the people served. Quality of life is essentially the extent to which we have the *freedom* and *opportunity* to experience life enrichment, to grow as human beings and create our own happiness, and to feel good about ourselves. We are motivated toward increasing our quality of life to the extent that we feel in control of our lives.

Active/Independent vs. Passive/Dependent

It appears to me that the major difference (affecting motivation for involvement in life and activity) between the active/independent person with a good sense of self-worth and personal control over his or her life, and the passive/dependent person is *focus*. The focus of the active/independent person is on maximizing positive experiences, enjoyment, and discovery. This leads to expanded living, positive risk taking, and reaching out to others.

However, the focus of the passive/dependent, hurting person is on minimizing pain. This leads to constricted living and the continued perceived safety of passivity. In effect, the passive/dependent person with a self-image of "patient" at times seems to be saying to us, "I dare you to make me happy," "I dare you to really care," "Go ahead, make my day."

Behind this frustrating attitude or behavior is the most basic motivation that keeps all of us from getting involved—*fear*. This can include:

- fear of pain, loss, or rejection;
- fear of what others will think;
- fear of wasted effort;
- fear of meaninglessness or disappointment;
- fear of being used;
- fear of looking foolish or childish;
- fear of poor performance or failure;
- fear of being ignored; and,
- fear of embarrassment.

With all this fear floating around inside a person telling him or her not to get involved, what can you as a therapeutic recreation leader do?

Your main role as therapeutic recreation leader and caregiver is that of a catalyst—something which stimulates action. People respond, to a great extent, to what we expect of them. If we expect a person to be incapable, dependent, and passive, he or she will quickly learn how to play these roles. However, if we expect them to have some ability and responsibility in making decisions about their life based on various options (that we might point out to them), then they may attempt to show some initiative, given the circumstances of their condition. For better or worse, the expectations of others can have a powerful effect on how a person defines himself.

Motivational theorists have generally agreed that "both internal factors (sometimes termed 'drive') and external factors (usually termed 'incentive') jointly determine motivation" (Toates, 1986).

As an effective helper, you must promote self-motivation in the individuals with whom you work—motivation to become reinvolved in life to the best of their ability, as well as external incentives. This can only be done if the messages received are messages of realistic hope along with the reestablishment of some sense of personal control over their lives. This is why providing choices can be so important.

You are the person giving these messages. You are the one who tells another, by your behavior, attitude, and expectations, that he or she is supported in a quest for personal empowerment. You are the one who must allow this other person to seek and find happiness on his or her own terms, and to make changes necessary to bring this about. In many respects, only to "do for" is to really take away another person's right to independence.

This book will demonstrate what I have found to be the most effective techniques for moving an individual or group towards greater involvement in life activity, thereby increasing personal empowerment and quality of life.

Chapter 2

What Do They Really Need From *Me*?

Reflective Thought
Bill died the other day. He was just an old man in a nursing facility. An old man who liked football and was always glad to see me when I came down the stairs. An old man who spent his last days in a small, darkened room with a television set running constantly, a friend in the chair next to him, and two women who made repetitive sounds, hugged dolls and were incapable of intelligent conversation most of the time.
 Bill was another one-of-a-kind human being who came into my life briefly and disappeared suddenly without a chance for me to say good-bye. Maybe, just maybe, if we don't allow ourselves to hurt at the loss of an irreplaceable human being, then we will never really learn how to say "hello."

Probably the most difficult thing for new staff in helping professions to learn is that their technical skills are just a small part of what is needed by the people they serve. It would seem that some staff never learn this and stay stuck in mechanical roles.

Many end up looking for alternative benefits (e.g., money, power, status) to the original altruistic motivations that most likely led them to seek a helping profession in the first place.

We make a huge mistake if we lose track of the reality that to be an effective caregiver, we must always be willing to help others meet their needs, in addition to our own. This is as true in therapeutic recreation programming as it is in surgery or nursing.

I have observed that there seem to be several basic universal needs, especially of people in long-term care. These are need fulfillments that I think all people ask of caregivers:

Dignity

We all need to be treated with respect—respect for our individuality, respect for our interests and preferences, and respect for our values and opinions. A sense of dignity and self-worth is essential if a person is to be motivated towards involvement rather than withdrawal. Simply put, people will respond to you according to the way you treat them. Personal respect and dignity are not only their right, but are also your duty.

Affection

There is an exercise on loss that I do in my classes and workshops where participants are asked to quickly jot down ten of their favorite activities. They are then instructed to cross out anything they couldn't do or wouldn't feel like doing if certain conditions existed in their lives. One of the directions given is to cross out anything they wouldn't feel like doing if they did not receive any affection. It is amazing how much our motivation for life is diminished by the loss of daily affection. We simply need genuine hugs, pats on the back, and gentle touch for stimulation and a sense of togetherness. Although touch is most direct, affection can be shown with a kind word or a positive observation: "You got your hair cut. It really looks nice."

Once, while working in a long-term care psychiatric facility, I got into the habit of giving my clients a good-luck hug when they were discharged from the facility. It soon became obvious that others, who had not been assigned to therapy with me, were coming to my area and announcing when they were being discharged. Many of these clients would ask for a hug. Affection is vital to adding quality to our lives. Don't leave home without it. Do remember to *ask first* before touching a client or resident. Ask if he or she would like a hug. This gives him or her control over the touching and makes it safe. Remember that each individual has his or her own level of comfort with touching and affection. Be sure to respect individual differences and honor residents' wishes.

Sense of Control

This is essential to moving someone from a passive role to an active role. The key here is providing choice and respect for preferences. We need to feel that we have some control over our daily lives and what happens to us in order to be motivated to participate in life. We need to feel that our opinions and feelings will be respected and considered, and that we can influence others to a certain extent.

The learned helplessness that is prevalent in many long-term care facilities is simply the belief (perhaps based on the reality of the situation) that there is no control or influence over what happens. "The belief in helplessness is alleged to produce deficits in motivation and learning, negative affect" (Feather, 1982). It can have a drastic affect on the quality of one's life. We need to have choices in order to have a sense of control in our lives. Although too many (more than five) choices or options can be confusing, most of us respond positively to choosing between two or three alternatives. When working with residents who have a cognitive impairment, limit choices to two, simple, clear alternatives for best results. An effective technique is to offer a resident a choice between two activities (i.e., bingo or bowling) instead of a choice between attending or not attending. But, be sure to respect the resident's right to refuse both.

Stimulation and Challenge

For most people there is a need for stimulation, especially that which stimulates the senses and challenges our ability to think. (Yet, too much stimulation for some persons can be overwhelming and confusing.) Too often in healthcare facilities, staff automatically assume that other abilities are lost with the onset of whatever physical or psychological problem brought the person into the facility.

One staff member I know was thanked by residents in a psychiatric hospital for doing word games with them. The reason they were so grateful was that they were given a chance to think, something they said other staff didn't promote.

Perhaps the most effective lesson I was ever taught regarding the need for stimulation and challenge came from my first clinical supervisor in a long-term care facility. During the first week on the job I was ordered to go to a unit and just sit for four hours straight. I was not to leave, but just sit there and respond only if or when someone approached me. There was simply nothing to do, to look at, to pick up and manipulate, or to read—nothing to stimulate me to move. This proved to be four of the most depressing, frustrating, passivity inducing hours of my life, but I left that experience being forever acutely aware of the devastating effects of "nothing time" on personal motivation.

Usefulness and Meaninglessness

We all need to be needed and this seems to become more critical as we get older. We need to be reminded that our lives have not been lived in vain and that our presence is still useful. It is what keeps us going, what keeps us moving and participating in life. One of the most common statements heard from an older person with depression is, "I'm just not useful to anyone—nobody needs me." This is a belief that you, as an effective therapeutic recreation leader, must prove wrong constantly. You need to provide meaningful tasks that call for skills that are still intact, that fulfill the need to be needed, that provide a sense of purpose and usefulness. Especially with the elderly, this is an essential motivator for continued life involvement.

Chapter 3

Natural Motivators

Every truly effective therapeutic recreation program I have ever known has had as one of its components the purposeful enhancement of life enrichment skills. What are life enrichment skills and why are they such great motivators? These life motivators are the day-to-day good things that come our way, at least occasionally, from other people, from nature and animals, from children, and from our faith. These are the things that really add quality to and enrich our lives. They give us wonderful feelings and memories. And they can be the best part of living.

Let's look at some examples:

Wonder

Do you remember how stimulating and exciting discovery was when you were in the process of unfolding a mystery? Do you remember your first visit to a zoo, science museum, or aquamarine exhibit? Do you remember saying, "Oh, wow!" or, "I wonder how they got that way?" Discovery—that sense of wonder at or about something—can have a highly motivating effect on our lives. It wakes us up and calls us to awareness of what is fascinating in life.

This leads us to the next natural motivator.

Awareness

As people get older or are placed in a passive, "patient" role, they can begin to shutdown emotionally, to lose their sense of awareness. For a person who finds it traumatic or unbearable to be placed in a long-term care facility, this dissociation can be a survival skill, blocking out the unbearable. We must be aware that it can also greatly decrease the quality of his or her life. In shutting down the awareness of what is negative in life, a person will also tend to shut down awareness of what is good, pleasant, and positive.

You, as an effective motivator, need to make people aware of the good things. For example, you may need to even point out to someone that he or she seems to be enjoying himself or herself because he or she is laughing. Your own awareness of what your senses are perceiving and the sharing of those perceptions is important in helping others become aware again. This will be discussed further in Chapter 4.

Gentleness

This seems to have become a lost art with the constant time demands that are placed on caregivers. When we feel rushed, there is a tendency to be curt and to appear uncaring. Gentleness comes from our ability to give our full attention and respect to each person *as* we are serving him or her. It comes from looking on each person with affection and realizing that neither of us will be exactly the same again. It also comes from the ability to realize that this moment, and not what we intend to do next week, is life. If you can gain the ability to live in the moment and behave as the person you would like to be, in that moment, you will discover an increased sense of respectful gentleness that contains much strength.

Appreciation

This is a life enrichment skill that the elderly population have mastered especially. The act of *being appreciated* can be highly motivating. The simple act of saying "thanks for joining us," or "I really appreciated your help with that program," or "I love it when you smile because your eyes seem to sparkle" can have a powerful effect on motivating someone to get involved again. Most of all, just be sincere.

Curiosity and Anticipation

These are wonderful motivators because they give us something to look forward to, to hope for, and to wonder about. Build up your programs with anticipation ahead of time and you will definitely have more people attend. Give people a sense that something special is going to happen. Make them curious. Then make it special.

Being Listened To

To have someone's full attention is a rare gift and can be a highly motivating and energizing experience. When you have given me your full attention and have allowed me simply to be me without judgment or expectation, I become more open to trust, more open to what you have to say and what you have to offer. Being listened to validates a person's uniqueness and allows for a greater, more comfortable involvement in life's activities.

Other Motivators

Anytime you offer someone the chance for *enjoyment, creativity, humor, spontaneity, hope,* and *exhilaration,* you offer a life enriching experience and a natural motivator. And anytime you offer someone *kindness,* you offer what I feel is perhaps the greatest natural motivator. Sincere, genuine kindness (i.e., born out of respect rather than pity) is perhaps the highest expression of caring. It is also a wonderfully effective way to gently urge someone to respond to life.

Section II

Chapter 4

Practical Motivators

Well, here they are, some of the best, most effective motivators for getting people to say "yes" to involvement in therapeutic recreation programs and life in general. Some you may have discovered yourself, others may be new to you, or something might spark a new idea for you. Just keep trying to add to your skills as a motivator and you will gradually become increasingly more effective at providing quality service.

The Therapeutic Recreation Process

The Therapeutic Recreation Process consists of four steps: assessment, planning, intervention and evaluation (APIE). As you read through the following suggestions of practical motivators, think of how each can be used throughout this process. First, in the assessment phase, gather information you need to decide on which motivators you want to try with each resident. You might want to use a checklist for this purpose (see Figure 4.1, page 18). Second, you may want to build them into your goal plan and approaches as well as program planning. Third, each of the motivators is implemented in the intervention phase. Be sure to document which were used in your progress notes and the results. Finally, in the evaluation phase, keep track of which motivators work for each client and which ones don't work. By keeping this therapeutic recreation process focus, you can incorporate these motivators into your overall therapeutic recreation program.

18   Getting People Involved in Life and Activities

Make Brief, Frequent Contact

I have found this to be the best technique for motivating people for eventual participation. The more someone is exposed to consistent, positive contacts with another person, the easier it is to trust that person. People who are living in long-term care facilities, especially the elderly, can easily be overwhelmed by interactions that are too long in duration or too demanding. When this happens, there is a tendency to simply shut out future social pressures. These brief, consistent contacts by you let someone know that you have been thinking of him or her without the expectation of further social demands. A person then feels noticed just for who he or she is.

Figure 4.1 Motivator Assessment Checklist

Name _____

Room # _____ Resident # _____ Date _____

Directions: Place an "X" next to a motivator that might be effective with this client.

☐ Brief, Frequent Contacts	☐ Fun
☐ Resident as Teacher	☐ Limit Alternatives
☐ Personalize Interaction	☐ Concrete Visual Cues
☐ No Demand Situation	☐ Humor
☐ Equal Chance to Win	☐ Utilize Strengths
☐ Program for Success	☐ Consistent and Truthful
☐ Inclusion	☐ Refreshments
☐ Ask for Help	☐ Staff Participation
☐ Get People Involved	☐ Spontaneous Reminiscing
☐ Use Props	☐ Stimulate Senses
☐ Be Someone Else	☐ Client Input to Activities
☐ Personal Invitation	☐ Staff Be Human
☐ Welcoming Environment	☐ Bridge Next Activity
☐ Enthusiastic Staff	☐ Teach Awareness
☐ Do What's Familiar	☐ Focus on Empowerment
☐ Special Events	☐ Assess Motivation Stages and Strategies
☐ Savor the Moment	

For those in long-term care rehabilitation settings who have communication difficulties, this can be a very effective technique. The frustration of trying to communicate is lessened by the brevity of the interaction, yet they are given the chance to socialize in a positive way.

I remember one woman with a severe speech impediment who was always sitting in the same place in the hallway of a nursing facility. Whenever I would pass by her I would "turn on" my nonverbal behavior. We could carry on wonderful conversations with our eyes, smiles, and gestures. My verbal messages or questions were calculated to allow for one-word responses. She would light up with animation when she saw me coming her way. My slight adjustment allowed her to actively participate socially without frustration. The brevity and frequency of the interaction was something that she could handle easily.

In the techniques of making brief, frequent contacts, the most important aspect is the sincere noticing of another person. You will find that he or she will look forward to your visit and what you have to offer, gradually hoping to spend more time with you. With your brief positive contacts, a person will be much more likely to get involved in what you are doing because the task will be connected to being with you—a pleasant experience!

Be An Inquisitive Student—Let the Resident, Patient or Client Teach *You*

Ask "wonder" questions such as, "Did you ever wonder...?" Don't be afraid to say, "Thanks, you just taught me something." People, especially older people, love to be helpful and in a giving role. It can be a very positive and therapeutic role and can immediately promote interest and involvement. Teaching another person stimulates one's mind, imagination, visual images, and memory; and it increases self-esteem. It is a great way to feel useful.

In a psychiatric setting, for example, it can be extremely therapeutic to help someone realize that he or she has something to offer to others. I recall one elderly depressed woman who had been lying in bed all day, showing no apparent interest in anything. Upon discovering that she had been an ardent indoor gardener at one time, I asked her if she would mind giving me some advice on care of the plants in our Hobby Center. By giving her the role of "consultant" I was able to get her actively involved in life again. Not only did she get out of bed to see the plants, but she continued to come on a daily basis to check on them until she was discharged. Because she was given a meaningful role, she regained a sense of usefulness and purpose and was able to get on with life in a more positive way.

The combined hidden knowledge, skill, and talent within the people you serve is much more extensive than you may realize. There is a strange tendency to limit people as a whole in our minds when we see them limited in a particular physical or mental sense. In doing this, however, you can miss sharing wonderful wisdoms and witticisms, along with truly enlightening learning experiences.

Every individual that you encounter has something to teach you. Don't be afraid to ask a person if he or she has ever participated in a particular activity or known someone who has. In a group, for example, simply to ask, "Has anyone ever...?" can stimulate motivating memories. Of course, you can then follow this up with the questions, "What was it like?" or "What did you learn from that experience?"

Have you ever noticed how good you feel when someone from out of town asks you for directions to a place that you know? Most of us are glad to have the knowledge and to be able to pass it on to strangers. When you create a situation which allows another person to teach you something, you put him or her temporarily in that role of a rescuer who has knowledge to share. It is a vital leadership role that can help a person feel useful. And, of course, when we human beings feel useful, the natural inclination is to want to do more.

Personalize Each Interaction

Use an individual's name (i.e., the one they wish to be called) frequently when you are talking to or referring to them. It's important that you do this casually at the beginning or end of statements. For example, you might simply say, "How are you feeling today, John?" or, "Mrs. Smith, would you please hand me the scissors?" Sounds simple, but it is surprising how many staff in facilities forget to use a person's name, thereby decreasing his or her individual dignity.

An easy way to feel comfortable with doing this is to start consciously using a person's name at the end of an answering statement. When someone asks you a question, simply end your answer with their name: "I plan to post the activity calendars this afternoon, Mary."

Someone once said that one of the most pleasant sounds we hear is that of our own name being spoken. If said in a positive way, it catches our attention and wakes us up. It can be wonderfully individualizing and dignifying to hear ourselves referred to by name, particularly if it is the name we wish to be called.

Remember also, that to some people a nickname can be very important to his or her identity. For example, if an elderly man has been called "Butch" or "Bud" all his life, and relates to that nickname, the formal "Mr. Jones" used all the time can be alienating and offensive to his identity. What's wrong with asking someone if they have a nickname they prefer that you use? Naturally, you might want to switch to their formal surname when communicating with other staff in team meeting situations or during other staff related business.

An important part of this motivational technique of personalization is a courtesy that is often overlooked. Many times, especially in long-term care facilities, we forget to introduce people to one another. We make the mistake of assuming that because we know who everyone is, they know who everyone is. Unless you know for sure, it is important to ask if people have met each other or know each other by name.

Although someone may recognize another person as the lady in the room across the hall or the man who sits in the wheelchair by the door, he or she may not necessarily know that person's name—or remember it. Consequently, socialization is minimized.

A person is motivated to become involved when he or she feels comfortable with those around him or her. A big part of this is personalization of each individual in a positive way by you.

Create a No Demand Situation

Ask someone to join you or the group, perhaps only as an observer. Let him or her know he or she will not have to perform or do anything unless he or she wants to. Most people are afraid to try new experiences because they don't know what will be expected of them in terms of performance. They are afraid of failing or looking foolish. With a no demand situation it is easier to decide to get involved. This passive participation is one of the easiest ways to begin to get someone involved in activity.

Think about the last time you attempted an activity for the first time or went to a social gathering or group meeting for the first time. Do you remember standing back and just watching or staying on the fringe of the group? This is natural acclimating behavior. Why should we expect more from someone we are trying to motivate for involvement?

If you are working with people who have chronic psychiatric illnesses, this can be a very important and effective tool for social involvement. As you know, social situations can be extremely difficult for someone with schizophrenia, for example. To allow that person a chance to participate without immediate social demands or expectations can be the first step to active involvement later.

There are many low demand roles that can be given to people that reduce the stress of a social situation. You can ask someone to be scorekeeper in a game or to serve refreshments behind a table. Counting or sorting things, observing others, passing out items, or collecting and putting away supplies at the end of an activity can all be low demand, yet participatory roles.

The important element in this technique is to create an atmosphere where there is no expectation or only low expectation of skill or social performance. Ideally, you should give the message that all you wish is the other person's presence with no strings attached at whatever therapeutic recreation experience you want them to attend.

This can be an excellent early motivational technique for someone who is depressed and has a low energy level. It is also very useful with those who are afraid of new experiences or the prospect of having to learn something new, as well as with those who may be overwhelmed by perceived physical limitations.

In effect, by using this technique, you are saying to people, "Come see what we have to offer. Simply watch and see if you like it. If you want to join in, great! But if you don't, I'd just be glad to have you there."

Provide a Fair Chance to Win

This is the basis of the ever-popular bingo or lottery. It is also why door prizes are a popular motivator. People want to be lucky and have hope that their chances are as good as the next person's for being rewarded. When the odds are stacked against us or any kind of favoritism is shown, we tend to withdraw from participation.

Ironically, if the odds are stacked against everyone equally, there is less of a tendency to withdraw. The lottery is a perfect example of this. Despite overwhelming odds of not winning when a lottery ticket is purchased, and repeated experiences of losing, many people habitually and almost religiously continue to purchase tickets. Hope still seems to "spring eternal"—when everyone feels they have an equal chance for success, and even more so when the odds are greatly reduced. Think of the last time you won something. Anything. I know you have—won something, that is—even if you need to think back to the coloring contest you won in the local newspaper, or the packet of seeds or pen that came in the mail. Wasn't it kind of special...just a little? Didn't you feel somewhat special, at least temporarily?

It's usually a pleasant experience to be given something free and to be labeled a winner. And the hope of winning either the item or the title can be a great motivator.

An equally important aspect of this technique is something that falls well within ethical boundaries—the equal distribution of goods. By this I mean that it is necessary for you to see that no favoritism is shown even when there is no contest or group situation. Everyone should be treated fairly and with equal regard.

Yes, it is easier to like some people more than others, but if you want to attract participants, they need to believe in the fairness of what you have to offer. This is especially true if what you are offering is tangible. So, when prizes, refreshments, supplies, and donations are designed to be given out in group activities, be sure not to pass on extras to particular people. This type of fairness may seem obvious, but it can be easy to forget, risking the trust you have built up in others.

Giving people a fair chance to win or receive something enjoyable can be an excellent way to spark interest in at least trying an activity.

A Better Way—Program for Success

If you can help people be successful when participating in an activity, they will be more motivated to do the activity again and to try new activities. One way you can accomplish this is to use the principles of attribution theory when planning and conducting an activity. Many people refuse this type of activity because they never win. Since there may only be one winner per game, chances are there will be many more losers than winners in games based on luck.

When people succeed or fail at an activity they tend to look for the cause of their failure or success. This is called attribution. They attribute the success or failure to one of two kinds of causes. One type of cause is called an "internal attribution." Internal attributions are either ability or effort. For example, "I was successful because of my ability and my effort." The other type of attribution is "external." External attributions are luck, task difficulty, or environmental factors. For example, "I failed because of bad luck, bad weather, and because it was a very difficult task." In general, participants will feel more positive about an activity and themselves if they attribute success to internal factors and failure to external factors. Success increases motivation while failure can lead to decreased motivation and helplessness (Iso-Ahola, 1980).

When programming for success and increased motivation, follow these attribution guidelines:

1. Make sure the activity is based on ability and effort, not luck. This allows you and the resident to control success through adaptation of the difficulty of the activity. This way neither of you is at the mercy of chance. For example, bingo is based on luck while bowling is based on ability and effort. The better your ability and effort, the more you will succeed.
2. Use cooperative activities, not competitive ones. This way everyone is a winner, there are no losers.
3. Encourage internal attributions to promote success. If a resident succeeds, attribute her success to her ability and her effort. For example, "That was great, Elaine. You're very good at this, and you put a lot of effort into it!"

4. Use external attributions to minimize failure. If a resident fails, attribute the failure to bad luck, environmental factors, or task difficulty. Then, *always* decrease the difficulty of the activity (i.e., move the target closer) and encourage the resident to increase his effort and try again. Be sure to adapt the activity so the resident will be sure to be successful. For example, "Oh, Bob, that was a stroke of bad luck. The carpet in here is not very good for bowling. Let's move a little closer and try a little harder!"

Motivate by Inclusion

Give each person a name tag, assign people to small task groups, or identify each table where people are sitting. Allow for even temporary team spirit to promote participation. Unless a person has mastered a skill, motivation will tend to increase if responsibility for performance is spread out among others as in a team.

Generally we like to be identified with a group, especially a winning or positive group. The concept of team spirit continues throughout our lives and this can be a great motivator for those who are participating only marginally.

Sometimes just a name that has been given to or selected by a project group can increase participation. Have you ever noticed how proudly some people will say, "I'm a member of the XYZ Sewing Club," or "I belong to the ABC gourmet cooking group"? There is a sense of team spirit and belonging that goes with being identified with others for a common purpose. This works on a temporary basis as well. It doesn't have to be a long-term project.

Watch interest increase when you temporarily identify people as a subgroup of a larger group activity, e.g., referring to "those at table 3" or "men vs. women." Almost immediately that basic tendency to want to be identified as a member of a group can be sparked. The spirit of camaraderie takes hold and interest is raised. A basic need of belonging is satisfied.

I have found that, when utilizing this motivating technique, it is better to try to place one or two people who are good at performing the activity with one or two who may not be able to perform especially well at that particular activity. For example, arrange a word game or crossword puzzle by group or table of people with varying abilities; or at a sing-a-long, try having staff or volunteers who enjoy singing or humming sit with those less active. Try to keep the focus cooperative, not competitive.

Ask For Help

This is probably the best immediate motivator, especially when working with the elderly. I have rarely, if ever, been turned down when asking for help with an activity or task.

Caution here: it is extremely important that what you are asking help with is a real need and that your request is sincere. We all want to be needed but nobody wants to feel manipulated or patronized. Also, make sure that what you are asking assistance with is within the individual's capabilities, so that he or she is successful with his or her assistance.

Finally, be sure to offer a choice when asking, "Would you like to help me with this activity?" so that the resident doesn't feel obligated or coerced into doing something he or she doesn't really want to do.

On numerous occasions I have been able to get through to someone who had given up on life by simply asking for their help. To stimulate your thinking, the following are some activities with which you might ask assistance:

You might ask someone to:

- hold something,
- count items,
- look for something in a magazine,
- take care of something for you (e.g., a plant),
- help prepare for an activity,
- cut up pieces of cloth for a craft project,
- help decorate a room or a cake,
- help bake cookies,
- help another person (e.g., someone who may need a reminder or even a friend),
- help serve refreshments at a program,
- take a survey,
- do an interview with someone (e.g., resident of the month, employee of the month),
- help fix something (especially effective with elderly gentlemen but make sure you follow all safety and risk procedures),
- be a consultant on something and give their advice,
- lead a group or call bingo,
- help give a lecture,
- help cut up vegetables,
- help remind you of something when they see you,

- make a list of items, ideas or needed supplies,
- greet people as they come into an activity,
- take care of a pet,
- water plants in the activity area,
- write something, and
- help plan programs.

The list could go on and on. I'm sure you can come up with even more creative ways of getting someone involved using this technique. It is an extremely effective first step to getting people to focus outside of themselves. Just be careful to initially ask something that is within the scope of easy achievement and skill.

Get People Involved With Each Other

By sharing with others or assisting one another, focus is taken off negative self-involvement, preoccupation with problems, and personal loss, all of which are demotivators to getting involved in life. You might ask someone to bring a friend to a program or to share a magazine when he or she is finished with it. You could ask one person to remind another about an activity program, which would promote communication. There is a tendency among people living in long-term care situations to isolate themselves from the people around them. Interaction can easily become limited to response to staff inquiries in these facilities.

However, we all have a need to feel affiliated with one another in a positive way. We want to feel connected, not only by group identification, but also with people in our lives we call friends. Friends and acquaintances give us reasons to communicate and become involved in life and activities. We tend to do many activities, especially social activities, that we probably wouldn't initiate on our own, because of our friends and acquaintances.

If you look at your own life, you will realize that there have been numerous times when you decided to do something only because someone else, a friend perhaps, asked you. I have observed that this phenomenon tends to hold true for us throughout our lives. You are much more likely to get involved in something if a peer asks.

Likewise, a person is more likely to become involved or continue involvement in an activity if he or she feels he or she is doing it for a friend or because he or she is needed to help finish something. So, you might find it more beneficial to ask two people to do a project together if you think they will work well together.

I have found that for this technique to be effective with people who may have lost their natural socialization skills, you need to be very specific about what you want them to do or what you request of them. For example, instead of simply asking them to bring a friend, you might say, "Millie, when you come to the next activity program, would you mind asking Ann if she would like to come with you? I think she would like to participate if she had someone to go with her."

Even if Ann refuses to come to the program, at least the stage has been set for further interaction between the two of them. By creating realistic opportunities to communicate socially, you give people a chance to continue to maintain their social skills and to feel socially responsible. And this increases the likelihood of further personal involvement.

Use Props

Have you ever noticed what happens when the average person enters a social situation such as a party or group meeting? They find a "prop," something to hold or manipulate in their hands. It can be a drink, a cigarette, or a pen. Whatever the object is, the result is usually the same. Props tend to reduce social tension and can have the added effect of increasing imagination by changing a person's image or role. This is why you will probably get a better movement response from someone exercising with a Fred Astaire top hat and cane, for example.

Props allow us to be someone other than who we are or other then how we see ourselves. We can become instant actors with a prop; our imaginations are stimulated, and our inhibitions are temporarily forgotten. Think about what you might do if I were to hand you a sword, a pair of drumsticks, or a kitten. Assuming you weren't allergic or fearful of the kitten, you would most likely start to play naturally with each of these. You would, in effect, become naturally involved in something outside of yourself.

Props can provide wonderful stimulation for people who have become nonverbal for various reasons. They allow us to communicate with our environment and each other in a nonverbal way. They can serve as a stimulator for creative imagination throughout our lives, provided the props are things we can relate to in a positive way.

Of course, when you use props, be sure that they are age-appropriate. No one wants to feel childish by being handed something that he perceives as a toy made for children. So if possible and safe, use the real thing when you use props in therapeutic recreation programs. An example of this could be the drumsticks I handed out before. I wouldn't give plastic, play drumsticks or ones that had been painted with primary colors. I would give a real set of drumsticks. Another example is party decorations. It is appropriate to have party hats, streamers, and noisemakers for a New Year's Eve Party. However, the same type of party hat might be inappropriate at a birthday party for an elderly person.

There is another caution when using props to motivate. Be sure to hand someone something that you think he or she will be able to manipulate successfully. To be a motivator, the prop must be viewed as being meaningful in some way and providing a positive outlet for expression. If one feels foolish or cannot manipulate the drumsticks successfully, it can have the reverse effect and be a demotivator. Being given something that is too difficult to manipulate can keep that someone from getting involved the next time. One suggestion is to supply a large basket or cart with props, allowing participants to choose.

Props can be great motivators on a temporary basis. Ironically, in this case you need to give some prior thought to creating an atmosphere in which spontaneity can occur.

Allow People To Be Other Than Who They Are

This is a sequel to the technique mentioned above. It is a technique that allows people to get out of their perceived limited life roles and to act as if they were more than their mind tells them they are. It can be done through costumes, dress up, role-playing, creative drama, or skits. Just be sure the activity is appropriate to their age.

Creative imagination is enhanced and social stress reduced when we are allowed to be other than who we are perceived to be at times. It's almost like taking a cork out of a bottle and letting the juices flow. We feel free and uninhibited when playing the role of someone else.

As a professional counselor, I once had a client call me on a weekend in a temporary crisis. During our conversation she stated, "Tomorrow when I go to work, I'll be all right because I can play a role and be someone else. It's today when I have to be me that is hard...."

Perhaps one of the most difficult and stressful tasks we have as human beings, is learning sincerely to love, respect, and live who we truly are—to be our genuine self. This type of personal integrity and congruity is rare, partially because few people seem to have sufficient self-esteem to feel comfortable just being themselves. We find it much easier and less stressful at times to act out our ideal self, the person we wish we could be. If a person is nonassertive in life, it is probably easier for him or her to play the part of an assertive person than to really be one.

I noticed this many times at Halloween dances where residents were allowed to dress up in costumes. Most of the time people seemed to choose costumes and characters that were opposite to their own daily personality and behavior. The costume seemed to provide an outlet for behavior and a role that would normally be difficult and stressful for them. Because of the play-acting, the energy level was much higher than usual, also. The freedom of the role greatly enhanced creative imagination and spontaneity.

Obviously, it is important to keep things in perspective and to make it clear that someone is only temporarily playing a role. And there are certain conditions or diagnoses with which you would want to exercise caution such as some forms of schizophrenia and dementia. You would not want to feed into a resident's delusions. It is also important that a person feels comfortable or expresses interest in taking on a particular role, even temporarily. But in general, it can be a fun and stimulating motivator to create a situation where people can get out of themselves for a little while and simply be someone else.

Give A Personal Invitation

We all want to be wanted and included, and one of the best ways to make others feel wanted is to ask them directly—to personally invite them—to join you. This is an extremely effective technique that is vital to the success of any therapeutic recreation program. Signs, calendars, and announcements are necessary but will never take the place of a personal invitation when it comes to getting someone to come to a program.

This request to do something makes a person feel special, similar to being asked to do a command performance. It enhances the dignity of the individual and creates a personal bond between you and the individual. Anytime you create a situation where another person feels special, you increase the chances of further communication and social involvement. Very simply put, when we feel better about ourselves, we are much more likely to get involved in things outside ourselves.

In my observations, I have noticed time and again that people would become actively involved in therapeutic recreation programs to the extent that they felt good about themselves. One of the ways to feel good about yourself is to feel special, to be wanted or needed, or to have someone look forward to your company. (Isn't that one of the feelings you have had as a caregiver?)

I have probably been more successful at getting people to come to therapeutic recreation programs by personally inviting them than by any other means. But once again I must caution you to be sincere. If you are not, you will be seen as a fake or a "con man" who just wants to increase attendance numbers. This will have the opposite effect, destroying any trust relationship and your ability to motivate in the future. Always be sincere in your interaction with those you serve. The elderly seem especially adept at recognizing those who fake interest in them.

In inviting someone to come to a program, be honest about why you want him there. If it's part of a care plan, it's all right to remind him. Even if you're not sure he will enjoy himself, say that. "Well John, I don't know (or can't promise) you'll like it, but I think it's worth the effort to try. I'd really like to see you there. I hope you decide to join us."

Don't give up on invitations when the first few are ignored. People may test you for awhile. They may even try to push you away or reject you. This may occur for several reasons and have nothing to do with you. Many times it is because others have given up on them in the past and this is expected of you also. Sometimes it happens because to say "No" is the only sense of control someone feels. Sometimes, because of the pain of experienced losses, a person is fearful of getting involved or liking another person again. It becomes easier not to care too much.

However, you will find that if you are consistent in a gentle, sincere, and positive way, you will go far toward getting even the most distant individuals to gradually come out of their shells. Even if they never decide to come to an activity program, their lives will have been enriched by your regular and encouraging interactions—your brief, frequent contacts. And increasing or enriching the quality of life is the ultimate goal.

Create A Welcoming Environment

Create a setting and atmosphere that supports the process you have planned. For example, if you want people to socialize, place chairs and tables in a way that will promote socialization. You may need to have long tables set up end-to-end for crafts, but this can be a terrible arrangement for a Resident Council meeting where you want people to interact, especially if some people have hearing impairments. A better arrangement would be to place the tables so that they form a square, making it easier for people to see and hear each other. You also might want to remove tables completely from the immediate activity area.

Also, eliminating or reducing distractions can be helpful towards increasing involvement. You might try turning off the background music, placing "Please Do Not Disturb" signs outside a room or a sign that indicates a special meeting is in progress. Environmental elements alone are so important that it would take another book in itself to go into all that is possible here.

One way to help make the atmosphere of an activity program or experience welcoming is to think about what you would do if you were having some friends or family over for the activity.

Ask yourself these questions:

- How would you initially invite them?
- How would you arrange the furniture?
- How would you greet them when they came through the door?
- How would you introduce those who weren't familiar with everyone?
- How would you initiate social interaction among those who didn't know each other well?
- How would you make everyone feel "at home"?

My point is that one of the best ways to have a welcoming environment in an activity program is to treat people as your guests, for this is what they really are—guests in your part of the world.

Another important element of this technique is to make your activity environment livable. Have you ever noticed how some houses you enter make you feel comfortable and free to either sit and relax or to move around and explore? This is the effect you want to create around an activity area. One of the ways to do this is to have selected items out and readily available for use. For example, people will probably not think to ask for a jigsaw puzzle, but if one is partially put together with the outside border finished, there is greater motivation for working on it.

The same concept applies for certain table games. When they are visible and readily accessible, the inclination to play is stimulated. Interest in taking part in a craft or hobby program is stimulated by seeing the end result displayed. And the possibility of someone planting something in a pot or garden is greater if the tools and potting soil are readily available.

The bottom line for those living in a long-term care situation is, if they have to ask for it, they probably won't think of it or won't want to bother you. But if the environment invites interaction, then motivation for involvement can be greatly increased.

Be Enthusiastic

Sounds simple enough, maybe even obvious, but it's amazing how many therapeutic recreation staff forget this most basic technique. We are drawn like a magnet to someone who is genuinely enthusiastic. We want to be in his or her company. We want to do what he or she does. We want to find out what it is that he or she finds so interesting.

You can be that magnet for others if you consciously try. The trick may be to see yourself as a professional performer with a "showtime" mentality. Do whatever it takes to turn yourself on in a positive way so that others will be attracted to what you have to offer. Take a cue from professional performers and consider what it is that gets your attention and maintains it (other than their talent). Doesn't part of the attraction come from the energy that you feel flowing in them? This type of showtime energy and mentality is what enhances enthusiastic behavior and creates that magnet effect.

Many times my enthusiasm has been intensified dramatically by just reminding myself that I had the opportunity and privilege of increasing the quality of life for a particular individual or group through my interaction with them. It's important to remind yourself of the potential impact you have on those you meet. They will respond to both your attitude and your energy level. And both need to be positive.

Perhaps enthusiasm is most effective when it focuses on the positive aspects of a situation. When you express enthusiasm for a program or project, concentrate on what is potentially good about it rather than what negatives it can eliminate. In other words, concentrate on what you perceive as the outcomes of the activity. This will aid you in expressing enthusiasm for the program or project. For example, you might say, "How about a good laugh—we have a comedy show tonight. Care to join me?"

Be sure that you believe what you are trying to promote and that it is something in which you would enjoy participating. Otherwise your performance will be seen as a sham and/or a manipulative ploy. After all, the best performers love what they do. Consequently, there is a sense of reality and genuineness that emanates from them. If you truly feel that what you have to offer is something meaningful and fulfilling (as it should be), then much of your enthusiasm will be automatic and natural. So, allow this natural love of life to show. We motivate by example much more than we realize.

Do What Is Familiar

People are much more likely to get involved in something that is familiar to them rather then something where the expectations are totally unknown. They may not be able to do or perform anymore, but they will be more motivated to participate in a spectator role of something familiar. This is a good way to get people involved who are functioning at a lower level.

This technique can go hand-in-hand with the "ask for help" technique. If you ask for help from someone you know has mastered a skill at one time in his or her life, he or she will be much more likely to say yes to your request. People like to be seen and respected for their expertise and accomplishments. They feel privileged to have an opportunity to display their talents.

Don't overlook residual skills that have become second nature to someone simply because of the years involved in doing a particular skill. A man who has worked with his hands as a carpenter for 50 years may be more willing to get involved with an activity that includes hand tools. A woman who was head cook at an elementary school for 30 years might want to help plan, prepare, or serve refreshments.

Participation is increased when less effort is needed to perform a task. This is true of us all, but seems especially true of many elderly people in long-term care facilities. If you can decrease the amount of perceived effort in a task or project, you will probably be able to increase the individual's desire to participate. I am convinced that most table games that are left standing unused in activity rooms are unused because people simply don't want to bother reading the directions to learn how to play the games. This doesn't mean that people are lazy. It just means that they are less likely to initiate involvement in something unfamiliar to them.

If you display materials and supplies in a craft or hobby area, someone coming into the area may ask about a new hobby, but he or she will tend to pick up an activity with which he or she is familiar. Success is motivating. If we have been successful in the past with something, we will tend to repeat what we have mastered.

Many times I have been able to get someone who was feeling down or depressed involved in an activity by simply offering him or her something that I knew he or she was familiar with rather than asking him or her to make a decision. Sometimes a person will pick up an activity by rote participation. Only after becoming engrossed in it will he or she remember the enjoyment that came from it. This is similar to the old recreational therapy adage that "involvement precedes interest."

Make Programs Special

There is a lot that can and should be learned from the advertising field. Simple techniques can turn an ordinary activity program into a well-attended, professionally organized one. Yes, you need to advertise your services!

If people could satisfactorily plan their own leisure involvement at all times, you would not be needed. So don't be afraid to borrow motivating techniques that have proven to be effective at getting attention. Some of my best programs were augmented because of the use of phrases and/or conditions like "limited time only," "this week only," or "limited to the first ten people who sign up." Look at commercials and see what catches your attention. It was not included by accident.

People want and need to look forward to something. Think about your last vacation or planned activity with friends. There is a good chance that one of the better parts was what took place before it—the looking forward to the experience. This experience of anticipation of something can be a wonderful motivator and can draw people into an event who would normally not get involved. It can create a positive social atmosphere that has people talking and focusing on the expected pleasurable experience. It can create a "you-don't-want-to-miss-it" atmosphere that increases a sense of community and oneness.

One way that advertisers do this is to create a sense of mystery or anticipation about something. "Coming soon!" is an example of this. A countdown to the big day or special event can also help. You might try using a special color with all advertising for the program, so that when people see that particular color, they immediately associate it with enjoyment and the program.

Try augmenting a special event program with other subprograms that relate to it. You might invite people to help prepare refreshments for the big event or to make door prizes or costumes. If you are planning a special trip, you might want to have a program that discusses or teaches something about what the participants might see or do.

This technique applies mostly to special event type therapeutic recreation programs and the emphasis is on going all out to promote interest. It can be equally appreciated, however, when regularly scheduled programs are enhanced by an occasional surprise that is enjoyable to the participants. Some homemade refreshments served during a program that normally doesn't have food can be a pleasurable surprise. (Of course, you would need to follow all medical and dietary protocols.) Little surprises such as this can change what has become routine into something special, more relaxing, and even memorable.

Provide Something That Helps Participants Savor the Moment

This could be a picture, a favor, or anything that will promote memory of the activity. One of the most popular requests I have received occurred when I casually offered to take one person's picture with the therapeutic recreation department's resident cat. One by one, as word of mouth spread, individuals would come to my office asking if they also could have their picture taken with "Patches." This unplanned activity seemed to provide a simple link to the continuity of life and the creation of a new memory.

There are so many negative reminders in the environment that can bring a person down. These can be anything from the consistently cloudy weather, to the rude and brusque interactions of certain staff members at a facility, to tasteless food, to therapeutic recreation programs that are demeaning and boring, or to simple loneliness.

Anytime you give people realistic hope or positive memories, you increase the quality of their lives. Let people see themselves actively living to the extent possible with their limitations. Remind them of the enjoyment they showed or expressed about an activity experience. This can be done with participation pictures that are given to them individually or posted on a bulletin board. (However, for this to be motivating, be sure the individual sees the picture as something positive and not just another reminder of loss of skill.) You can reinforce reminders of a successful, positive experience by asking at the end of an activity how or what was most enjoyable about the activity experience. Also, by referring back to a previous positive experience, you give people the chance to savor the memory of it. This can be done by saying to a group, "Do you remember when we...?"

These types of reminders let people know that, despite their physical, mental, or environmental limitations, they still can enjoy life and have happy memories. What a wonderful gift for you to give.

Always Include Some Fun

Adapt activities to emphasize the "fun" part. For example, consider what you enjoyed most about playing baseball. If most of you say batting/hitting, this, then, would be the "fun" part of the activity that we would want to emphasize. Always think in terms of adapting the familiar activity so that the fun part is included and repeated for everyone. We automatically did this when we were younger by taking turns hitting fly balls. Another example is the trivia game Trivial Pursuit. The fun part is answering the questions, so we once simplified the game by eliminating the board. Winners were declared when answers were correctly given in all categories and the tokens were filled with colored wedges. This simplified the game tremendously and emphasized the fun part.

Consider bingo for a moment. What do you think is the fun part of this activity? I'll give you ten seconds to think about this.... Well, it's the winning and the prizes, isn't it? OK, even if you don't agree for some reason, let's assume this is true just for demonstration. If winning a bingo prize is the fun part of the activity, then how could you make this a bigger part?

One way this was accomplished was to display the small prizes on an upright board. It took only a few minutes to make loops of masking tape, put them on the back of each small prize, and place the prizes on a large board so that they were visible while people were playing the game. This display somehow gave greater perceived value to the prizes, making selection and choices special. People could see which prizes were left to choose if they won the next game. A large "Prizes" sign was posted at the top. This easy adaptation seemed to make a popular activity much more interesting for the participants.

Focus on Empowerment

Enhance a resident's sense of control over his or her environment, others, and his or her own life through a program of empowerment. In a long-term care setting recreation and leisure activities present an excellent opportunity to provide choices and resident control over outcomes that are not possible in others aspects of the institutional environment. The essence of leisure activity is its perceived freedom and control. Follow these guidelines to enhance the resident's perceived control through recreational activities (Martin and Smith, 1993):

- assess and monitor perceptions of control in recreation activities using the Leisure Diagnostic Battery (Witt and Ellis, 1989),
- provide choices,
- develop decision-making skills,

- provide individualized activities based on needs and preferences,
- reduce or eliminate barriers to participation,
- be sure activities are age-appropriate,
- normalize activities and encourage community outings,
- provide opportunities for social interaction,
- include opportunities for spiritual development and creativity, and
- encourage active participation.

Give Choices, But Limit Alternatives

Too many choices can lead to confusion and a desire to withdraw from an activity. The effect of having too many choices and decisions to make at once is similar to the fatigue that can take place when shopping in a busy department store. We can become overwhelmed with too much stimulation, too many options, and too many choices. How many times have you heard someone in a restaurant ask for a recitation of the dozens of ice cream flavors available, only to finally decide on vanilla or chocolate? Decision making can be difficult. Most of the time people will choose something that is familiar and known to have a positive outcome in the past.

When you give limited choices, you allow a person to stay in control and not become overwhelmed. This is especially important for those who have dementia or other disabilities which interfere with the thought processes.

Limited choices can also be a good tool to use when there is a problem with inappropriate or manipulative behavior, as with people who have major psychiatric illnesses or personality disorders. Many times a person attempts to test limits (i.e., the rules), partially to see how consistent and safe you are. When asking this person to change his or her inappropriate or unacceptable behavior, it can be very effective to give him or her two alternatives. This allows the person to save face yet be responsible for his or her behavior. For example, you could say, "John, you can either stop (doing that) or you can return to your unit. It's your choice." (Be sure you are prepared to follow through.)

With so little sense of control and so few options available, especially to people living in long-term care situations, the opportunity for choice can be very motivating. Choices are essential to a quality therapeutic recreation program, but you will find greater motivation if they are limited to two or three at a time.

Give Concrete Visual Cues

We are motivated to get involved when we are tuned into what is happening and know what is expected of us.

Visual cues constantly orient us in our environment, often without our being aware of them. They keep us in constant communication with our immediate surroundings. Traffic lights tell us when to stop, go, or slow down. Weather symbols in the corner of our TV screens caution us about impending tornadoes or floods. And who hasn't entered a new restaurant without looking for the restroom signs.

These visual cues help to reduce confusion and provide an easier transfer from one environment to another with less disorientation. The cues, of course, need to be accurate.

Once when I was visiting a nursing-care facility as an Ombudsman, I was stopped by one of the residents who pointed to an activity calendar and said, "They think we're stupid and we're not. I know that it's November and not October." Sure enough, it was November, but the large calendar listing all of the activities for the month was labeled October at the top. Although this lady was not thrown by the oversight, I wonder how many others were naturally confused about the Thanksgiving dinner being held in October.

You utilize visual cues every time you put up a sign of any kind, make a display, or choose colors to decorate a therapeutic recreation area. These cues are designed to sell and to motivate. But to do so effectively, they must be well-planned. (Have you ever confronted a bulletin board that was overcrowded and had outdated messages on it? After awhile, you just avoid looking at the clutter and misinformation.)

When doing an activity, especially if you are teaching something new, it is important that you show what you are talking about. Demonstrate movement or skills that are required. Hold up an example of what a finished craft project might look like. Use color coding consistently so that people don't have to guess what the colors might represent. Use high contrast colors on signs so that they are easily read. Avoid pastel colors and use of highlighters on signs. Also, thicker/wider letters are easier to see than thin, large letters.

Visual cues can turn a drab, boring environment into something interesting and exciting, or they can help to create a sense of peace and calm. The potential to stimulate is endless. Use them carefully and consistently, and you will be amazed at how effective they can be.

Use Humor and Laughter Often

Laughter is naturally therapeutic, both physiologically and psychologically. It is a natural stress reducer and social enhancer. We simply feel better when we laugh. Humor is a great motivator because it leaves us wanting more at a later time. And it counteracts all the negative influences that are inherent in our daily lives.

This is even more true for the people you serve since the negatives can far outweigh the positives in their lives.

Some specific ways of including humor in your programs are to:

- set up a cartoon bulletin board or scrapbook.
- include jokes and even riddles in your facility newsletter.
- share jokes that you recently heard with those in your programs. These can be introduced by saying, "I wonder if you've ever heard this joke?"
- set up a situation where people can watch the antics of children, puppies, or kittens. This always brings on smiles at the very least, and usually genuine laughter.
- include some of the old comedy routines that would be well-known to us all, but especially familiar to the elderly.
- become aware of and point out naturally funny things that happen during the day. (Of course, you need to make sure this is not done in a way that "makes fun" of another person. No one would want to be the subject of your joke.)

Don't be afraid to laugh at yourself, in a kind way, of course. We all need this for balance and perspective. And when others can see your ability to not take things so seriously, it can become easier for them to lighten up a little and focus more on the positive.

Humor is a good motivator for future participation. We all want to be where there is laughter and fun. This condition is best created with healthy, wholesome, and natural humor that does not include "put downs" of any kind. Open yourself to the natural humor in life and you will have more to share with others.

Utilize a Person's Strengths

Let someone know that you recognize his or her talents or special skills and ask him or her to share them in a specific way. A person is much more likely to participate in something that has been done well previously, in a skill that has been mastered.

This is one of the most overlooked areas when an assessment or evaluation is done on a person entering a long-term care facility. As mentioned previously, for some reason there is a tendency to see the new resident as diminished, not just with his or her disability or condition, but as a whole person. And because of this narrow vision, we can miss really knowing the person as a unique human being with special talents, knowledge, and wisdom.

When you take the time to learn someone's special abilities, past successes, personal triumphs, and natural talents, you give honor and dignity to his or her uniqueness. And when you ask him or her to share these in a specific way which will bring further success, you provide the natural motivation of feeling needed and useful.

This motivating technique is somewhat like "Ask for Help" but the focus is different. When you ask someone for help, you are usually asking him or her for a favor from his or her perspective. When you set up a situation where someone can utilize his or her strengths, you allow him or her to share with and display to others a very positive part of himself or herself. (For example, you might feature a resident musician in a musical activity program.) Knowing that you have something special to share with your "community" can be a powerful motivator for active involvement. It can give a person one more reason for getting up in the morning when there seems to be few reasons to put in the effort.

Always Be Consistent and Truthful

What does truth and consistency have to do with motivating people to get involved in life and activities? Have you ever worked in a situation or been acquainted with people who were not consistent and truthful? Remember how you felt after awhile? Inconsistencies and lies in our communication with others lead to distrust, resentment, and withdrawal. All of these are demotivators. They create distance between people.

Simply put, it is important that what you say is what you mean and what you say you are going to do, you do. For example, if you tell a resident that you will take him back to his room when he wants to go, do it as soon as he asks. This will help him trust you.

Show that you care, don't just tell people how much you care about them. People will read your actions long before they believe your words. This is one of the things I quickly became aware of when working in long-term care facilities. I noticed that my interactions with people were always carefully watched by those in the surrounding area. At times I could almost feel judgments being made about whether or not I was someone they wanted to get involved with if I should come their way. I soon learned that I was being judged especially for my genuineness and congruity.

Sometimes a person will constantly refuse activity involvement. But you might notice him or her "hanging around" the doorway, eventually entering, then appearing to "run away" again. Be aware that he or she may be testing the waters. It is similar to running down the beach and putting a toe into the lake or ocean. Realize that when this person joins the group, it is one of the highest honors he or she can give you. Don't forsake the trust.

Your consistency and truthfulness will do more towards building trust than anything. It will allow someone to feel safe with you and to risk increased involvement.

Serve Refreshments at the End of a Program

It is important to have something specific and concrete to look forward to in order to maintain interest. Unless it would be more appropriate not to wait because of the type of program, withholding refreshments usually serves to maintain the feeling that something enjoyable is still coming. I have found that when refreshments and prizes are not delayed, interest and motivation to participate can be quickly lost. This is especially true if you have participants who are functioning at a lower level.

This can also be true for particular settings. Staff working in long-term psychiatric settings quickly learn that they might lose their audience and/or participants if refreshments are distributed too early in the activity program. After eating (and smoking) some people may become restless or simply walk away from the program.

It seems to work best if you tell people at the beginning of the activity program when the refreshments, if they are part of the program, will be served. For example, you might say, "We're going to have (or do)...and.... Then we will be serving refreshments. Hope you enjoy the program."

This type of delayed gratification is a remarkable motivator for continued involvement. It is a promise of something that we perceive as assured enjoyment. People don't know for sure that they will like the program, but they know they will probably like the refreshments if they stay. By keeping the perceived "good stuff" until the end of a program, you create a situation where people leave on a positive note, also.

Yes, this sounds a little manipulative. But in terms of motivations for continued involvement, it is historically effective. Think about the contests that come in the mail and keep you involved by going from one level or step to another. "You have made the third round and are among those from whom our grand prize winner will come!!! But you must send back...." Well, you get the idea. Once again, what works in motivating you, will probably be effective (with adaptation) in motivating others. Delaying known gratification is one thing that commonly works.

Participate Yourself

Do this especially in small group activities. But be careful not to demonstrate a great discrepancy between the quality of your work and that of others. If you want people to be interested in something, they need to see that you find it interesting. Don't be afraid to share your interests and discoveries. As you participate, teach yourself and show the involvement you want from others.

This technique works well with hobbies and crafts. You will find that some people will get involved in order to demonstrate or show you different aspects of a craft which they remember from earlier years. Others will get involved because your participation gives them a demonstrable pattern to follow without having to read directions. Still others may get involved with the intention of wanting to encourage your efforts.

Many times I was able to stimulate participation by another person simply by combining my participation in learning how to do something with asking him or her to teach me, or by asking his or her advice when I got stuck. This can be effective especially when you have someone who has been successful in the past but is fearful of actively doing something now. Let's say you're working with a person who has had a stroke. Although he or she may not feel able actually to perform a certain task, he or she still may be willing to get involved in your participation in the task.

Perhaps the most effective aspect of this technique is the element of association. When you get involved in the therapeutic recreation experience, you are giving the message that it is meaningful and important to you and not just "busywork." You say, in effect, that this is something worth doing. And when you show that the activity is interesting or fun you create a visual as well as a verbal reason for participating. People would rather have fun with you than because of you.

Use Casual, Spontaneous Reminiscing

I have found that the best and most motivating time for reminiscing is while doing something else. This can be done with virtually any therapeutic recreation program, but seems to work best when you use it while working with either individuals or small groups. All you need to do is say something like, "You know, this reminds me of when...," or "Does anyone remember when...?" or "I wonder what it was like when...." Some of the most stimulating and motivating conversations can come from these casual references to the past. And this type of casual reminiscing can be much more effective at motivating involvement than a program which is specifically planned for it. It is a more natural and realistic way to reminisce.

Be alert to any small happening that could be used as a take-off point for pleasant memories. It could be a statement, the mentioning of an event, the performance of a task, a verse or melody in a song, or a picture. This type of link with the past is probably done in your everyday life with family and friends. Someone will say something and it will spark a memory. ("Do you remember when we...?")

When you create an atmosphere that allows for this type of casual reminiscing, you offer people a shared connection with the past, an opportunity to reexperience pleasant memories, and a link with the changes of today. It can be a very socially unifying experience.

Stimulate Multiple Senses

Create a situation where a person can become more aware of and relate to his or her own senses. Walk into a room and notice things. Point out what he or she may no longer see. Talk about how an object looks, feels, and smells. Make people aware of their surroundings. Give them something to hold. One way of doing this is to carry things with you as you visit people. Adopt the attitude of "Look what I found; I wanted to share it with you." It can be a freshly picked flower, a special texture (e.g., soft, silky), or a scent. A freshly baked cookie or muffin can stimulate wonderful feelings and memories.

Another awareness stimulator is to quietly ask, "Have you ever noticed...?" By asking a question such as this you help create visual images in the mind and turn on the sense of awareness. Sensory stimulation is well-known to those who work with people who have Alzheimer's disease or other forms of dementia. Utilizing it regularly can be very good therapeutic recreation programming. However, I feel the quality of the program can be enhanced if sensory stimulation is done in a more natural or casual way. The trick is to convey the impression that you are discovering or appreciating something yourself and asking the resident to join in your discovery.

Promoting sensory awareness can also be a great motivator with just about any population. Uses with children and those with developmental disabilities are historically well-known. In addition, I have used it therapeutically with psychiatric residents and with clients who have a history of physical or sexual abuse. Sensory stimulation is utilized automatically every time a floral arrangement or greeting card is sent to someone in a hospital or rehabilitation center.

When we have experienced pain or significant stress, for whatever reason, there is a tendency to shut down our feelings and awareness in order to diminish the pain. But this shutting down process, this attempt to make numb, is also likely to have a numbing effect on our sensory awareness. Consequently, we can lose out on the beauty of life and the hope that is needed in order to heal. When you promote the use of multiple senses, you help to bring people back to life or at least back to the awareness of life and the beauty that is in the world.

When you plan an activity experience or program, even if it is a one-to-one room visit, think about what you might do to stimulate the resident's senses in a positive way. It can help simply to remind yourself of the five senses: hearing, seeing, tasting, touching, and smelling. Try to think of something that utilizes more than one sense. For example, listening to music from the 1920s is one thing, but listening to that same music while looking at pictures from the same era utilizes two senses. If you add texture from fabric and the scent of lavender, you could stimulate additional senses. That's the idea and it can be done successfully with countless themes.

Many of the sensory stimulation theme packages that can be purchased commercially can also be put together by you with some thought and planning. Try taking a gallon size zipper-type, plastic storage bag and make up a sensory stimulation theme kit that can be used with individuals or in groups. Just pick a subject, such as "the ocean," and put items in the bag that represent or remind you of the ocean. You might have a cassette tape or compact disc of ocean sounds, a copy of the book *Gift from the Sea* (Lindbergh, 1975), a small bag of sand, some small sea shells, and a piece of driftwood. Get the idea? You could eventually develop a collection of sensory stimulation kits on various subjects for use in a variety of program settings. And they don't have to be in plastic storage bags. You could create various memory boxes each holding items surrounding one theme; items that can be held and manipulated, smelled and heard.

One word of caution regarding sensory stimulation. Often I have seen therapeutic recreation staff overdo this technique. It is possible to go overboard and provide too much stimulation.

This can irritate, tire, and confuse people who might have problems processing too much information. Aim for balance and consider the total environmental effect. For example, some programs, especially where there is discussion going on, do better without constant music in the background. Too many sensory distractions can make it difficult to focus on a subject. So be selective in the way you introduce things. Stimulate only one sense at a time, and only one stimulation of each sense at each session. For example, one smell, one sight, one touch, one taste, one hearing. If appropriate, additional sensory stimulation can be gradually introduced.

Utilize Their Ideas

Incorporate to whatever extent possible, any suggestions given by an individual or group. And then say "thank you" for the idea, even if you had to do a lot of revision to make the idea usable. People will become much more involved if they can see and experience the results of their influence and suggestions. Previously, I had mentioned how important it is for a person to feel he or she has some control over his or her life, to be able to make choices, and have what he or she says make a difference. This is one area in which you can bring this about and increase motivation for involvement at the same time.

One way in which this is, or should be, regularly done is through groups such as resident council committees in long-term care facilities, or other therapeutic recreation planning groups. But following through in some way with individual suggestions is equally important. You might try an activity program suggestion box, an interest survey, or a "best idea" contest. The goal here is not to get others to do your program planning for you but to give them a chance to have some influence over what is offered. (As an

Ombudsman, I have actually attended some resident council meetings where the therapeutic recreation director spent the entire time planning community trips for fewer than ten people when close to two hundred needed to receive service. Obviously, something was out of balance here.)

One of the best ways that I have found to utilize ideas is to pick up on comments that people make in passing. If someone states that he or she particularly likes a program, do more of it and let him or her know you remembered how much he or she enjoyed it previously. If someone takes delight in the memory of homemade muffins or real Italian pizza, see if this might be included in a cooking program and ask for his or her advice and involvement in the baking.

Sometimes just letting someone choose the colors for decorations or a display can enhance participation. Or if you know a person's favorite color, you could say "I was thinking of you, Martha, when I bought the pink table cloths for the picnic next week. I know it's your favorite color." This is an indirect way of making people feel they contributed and are special.

Allow Yourself To Be Human

Someone once said that "the main thing in life is not to be afraid to be human." In my experience, a major motivating factor in getting others involved has been my not being afraid to be human and to make mistakes. This has been especially true when it came to learning something new. It's important to allow people to relate to you as one struggling, sometimes laughable, human being to another. Yes, they need to see you make mistakes. But even more significant is how you handle your mistakes. What do you do when you spill something, forget a step in a process, or break something? How you respond to these mishaps can put things into perspective and teach others that there is nothing to be feared in trying.

We often take ourselves too seriously, holding on to unnecessary caution that can keep us from living fully. We're afraid of making mistakes and looking foolish or incompetent. But part of being human is the fact that we will fail at times, no matter how hard we try not to fail. If you can adopt an attitude that shows you are comfortable with both yourself and your lack of perfection, you can go far toward drawing people to you and what you have to offer them.

Don't be afraid to let some of your feelings show at appropriate times. Let people see your compassion.

Once I was doing an assessment (evaluation) of an elderly woman who appeared to be very depressed. As she started to walk away after the interview, I quietly said, "Mary, you look like you need a hug." The woman turned, literally fell into my arms and gave me a huge hug. She whispered in my ear, "Thank you so much! No one has touched me in years." Her husband had died years earlier, and I could feel the pervasive loneliness she had been carrying around with her. By recognizing and responding to her loneliness, perhaps her greatest need, the door was opened for reinvolvement in the social community and life in general.

There are times, of course, when you need to maintain boundaries from those you serve. But I have found that, in general, one of the best ways to get others involved in activity experiences is by just being myself along with my bent halo. To allow yourself to be human is to be someone who is nonthreatening and safe to be with—someone who is not playing a role or following a script.

Create a Bridge

...to the next activity, that is. Create a link from one program to another. Remind participants in one activity of what is coming up next, later that day, or tomorrow. Have you ever noticed how this is done on television? One show will plug an upcoming show or the show's hosts will say what is coming up in the next half hour. These are teasers that are meant to generate interest and a feeling of not wanting to miss something. And they do work. They keep you hooked or coming back for more. It's a way of saying, "If you liked this, wait till you see what's going to happen next!"

You can also create a bridge when you plan programs that feed into one another. For example, a crafts group that makes decorations for a special event or a cooking group that makes refreshments for a party, link together two separate but cooperative activity programs. These types of linkages provide a sense of community spirit and willingness to help that is essential to enhancing social interaction.

The trick is to get people with special talents involved in part of a bigger project or on successively linked projects. As they are working on one part of the project, talk about the bigger event and how what they are doing will make it better. For example, let's say you were planning to have an ice-cream social as a special event. You could have one program that serves as a planning committee; another activity could be a craft project that makes decorations to carry out the theme; and another activity could be for people who prepare the ice-cream topping; another group could help set up or serve. Meanwhile, everyone is talking about the upcoming ice-cream social. The more people are involved in various parts of a larger event, the more the excitement and anticipation, and the more likely they will be to participate in the larger event.

On a day-to-day basis, the bridging of one program to another can be a very effective motivational tool. Try making it a habit at the end of an activity program to thank people for coming, invite them back, and let them know that you look forward to being with them again.

Teach Awareness

Consistently refer to the good things in life. Point out beauty, goodness, nature, peacefulness, and kindness. As a specialist whose goal is to increase the quality of life for others, you are the catalyst for focusing their attention. You are the person in the best position to bring awareness of the good things in life back to those who may have lost their sense of wonder.

People are naturally drawn to someone who is consistently positive in his or her attitude. A huge part of maintaining this positive attitude is being able to stimulate your own awareness of what is good and beautiful in the world. This can be difficult to do in a world that seems to be focused on negative sensationalism. Everyday beauty and goodness seem to have a much less dramatic effect. But it is this fleeting awareness of what is positive that opens the door to daily doses of happiness and adds to the quality of our lives.

When you interact, demonstrating by example and pointing out to others what there is to be happy about, you give them a breath of fresh air that can breathe life into even the most faded outlook. To be most effective, this needs to be done casually without even mentioning the word happiness. By simply enhancing your own sense of wonder, you will automatically begin to share a feeling of excitement with others. Once I worked with a client who had a history of anhedonia (i.e., difficulty experiencing pleasure or enjoyment). I had taken her for a picnic lunch at a city park with a small lake. As we were sitting by a stream which ran from the lake, three Canadian geese flew by and made a simultaneous, perfect landing on the water directly in front of us. This was a scene I had viewed in pictures but to experience the real thing was breathtaking. My automatic and natural response was to exclaim, "Oh wow! Did you see that?!" I may not have been open to the magnificence of this scene had I not allowed myself to focus on the beauty of nature on previous occasions.

To help increase your own awareness, try the following suggestion: look at things as if you were seeing or discovering them for the first time. Look at them without judgment or evaluation of any kind. Open up your senses to the experience. Consider and picture in your mind some of the following:

- the tiny delicate moving fingers of a newborn baby;
- the clean-cut neatness of a freshly mown lawn;
- the sun striking a spider web in the morning dew;
- a six-week-old kitten at play;
- the silent soaring of a red-tailed hawk on a sunny day;
- the giggles of little children waiting with a pleasant surprise;
- a spontaneous hug from someone you love;

- the feeling of accomplishment after completing a difficult task;
- the smell of homemade bread, apple pie, or chocolate chip cookies baking in the oven;
- the shininess of a new toy or car (Remember getting new school or hobby supplies?);
- the warmth of a conversation filled with respect and affection;
- the softness of cuddling in a favorite blanket after being tucked in at night; and
- the taste of fresh strawberry preserves, a homegrown, just-picked, juicy tomato, or a homemade blueberry muffin still warm from the oven.

These are a few of the endless good things in life that can be relived in memory if not in actuality. You will find that once you start looking for and imagining a few of your own favorite things, you will be open to additional positives in your daily life. And this newfound awareness can be passed on and shared with others because your whole attitude and focus will have changed. We really do experience what we give our attention to and focus on. If you give your attention to positive things, then that is what you will increasingly experience and be able to pass on to others. You cannot share what you don't have to give. By focusing on an awareness of the good things in life, you enable yourself to share it with others. (They already know the negatives.)

Motivation Stages and Strategies

Motivation is seen as a process in which there are six stages. Each stage has a strategy that will help residents progress to the next stage. Assess your residents to determine where they fall on this scale, and determine the appropriate intervention:

1. In the *pre-contemplation stage* the resident is not aware of a need for change and doesn't want to do anything to change. For a resident in this stage, the best intervention is to give information and feedback about the problem to help the resident become aware of the need for change. Do not give suggestions or advice at this point. For example, "Evelyn, you look very sad and lonely sitting in here by yourself in your room" is feedback—how the resident appears to you. "You know, Evelyn, people who get out of their rooms and get involved in the activity program usually make out better than residents who don't" is information. Change the feedback and information during each visit, but keep reinforcing common themes.

2. In the *contemplation stage* the resident knows there is a problem, and is thinking about change. Usually she is going back and forth between pros and cons of changing. Evelyn may go back and forth in her mind: "I am sad and lonely sitting in this room, but I don't want to leave my room. I will sit here in my room if I want to, but do I really want to? I might not like those people, but if I stay in here I feel down." For the resident in this stage the best intervention is to find out what the resident is thinking and reinforce the side of change in a positive direction.
3. In the *determination stage* there is a specific window of time when the resident is open to change. The best intervention during this time is to help the client find ways to implement the change. Generate choices, explore options. Find ideas and evaluate them. For a lasting change, the resident will need to be successful, and have positive outcomes with the new chosen behavior.
4. In the *action stage*, the resident actually makes the change. He or she tries one of the options. In our example, Evelyn would attend an activity outside her room. The best intervention is for the change to be successful and enjoyable. Offer encouragement and support.
5. In the *maintenance stage*, once the person tries the change, the best intervention is to identify what the resident needs to do to maintain the change. For example, Evelyn might need a reminder of the time and location of the activity, assistance with transportation, or assistance in learning new skills needed in the activity itself.
6. It is best to plan for the *relapse stage*. Often the client will slip into relapse where she stops the behavior. The best intervention is to prevent discouragement and help her continue to think about change (Miller and Rollnick, 1991). For example, if Evelyn stops attending the activity, encourage her to think of other ways to get out of her room, such as a different activity or a better time to participate. Go back to stage three—determination.

This leads to a discussion of the biggest and most effective motivator—you!

Chapter 5

Their Greatest Motivation

Wouldn't it be great to have a cookbook that you could follow to create therapeutic recreation program menus and mix up social recipes that would instantly help people feel better? Wouldn't it be wonderful to be able to punch in a computer code that would instantly spit out the particular technique that is best to use with Mr. or Mrs. Smith? I certainly hope I am *not* predicting the future here. Because as easy as that might sound, mechanization and systemization such as this would lead us further away from quality of life rather than closer to it.

If you read (between the lines) about the techniques presented in this book you will find one common denominator—*you*. By far the best, most effective, most important motivator for getting the individuals you serve involved in life and activity is you! No one can ever give exactly what you have to offer. No one else will ever have your unique smile, your laughter, your sincerity, your ability to listen, your way of having fun, or your insight. No one else will ever be able to give the world exactly what you can because only you can be the best you that is possible.

I have discovered that people are most motivated to participate in life and activity to the extent that they feel good about themselves. Perhaps one of the greatest gifts that you can give to others is to create a situation where they feel good about themselves when in your presence.

The primary aspect of motivation is that it occurs in the relationship between the therapeutic recreation specialist and the resident. Carl Rogers (1961) outlines the helping relationship in detail. He states that the most important determinants of the quality of this relationship are the attitudes and feelings of the helper. Rogers feels that attitudes are much more important than any therapeutic technique. Unconditional positive regard is truly a gift that you can give a resident. To be accepted by another unconditionally is a real motivator.

There is an old Chinese saying that states, "Only happy people can make a happy world." There is much truth to this. Have you ever noticed that the people you feel safest with and with whom you want to spend more time, are those who appear to be happiest and most contented with themselves? They don't feel the need to compare or put down others, they're seldom negative, and they tend to concentrate on the good things in life. They seem to be basically happy and in control of and responsible for their own happiness. They have integrity, warmth, compassion, and gentleness. Yet you are impressed by their quiet strength and perspective on life. The hectic pace and tension of the day diminishes a little while in their presence. You feel better just being with them.

These people are rare, yet memorable. We want to be with them because we not only feel better in general, we tend to feel better about ourselves when we are with them. And when we feel better about ourselves, we are willing to get more involved in life. The more involved we become in positive life experiences, the more likely we are to do more.

Are you that quiet magnet that attracts people to the good things in life? Are you that unique person who can help others genuinely feel better about themselves? Are you the person they hope to see coming down the hall? Are you their biggest motivator for getting involved in activity experiences?

No matter how many cookbook techniques you learn and use, it is your sincere, open, genuine caring that will have the greatest impact on others. It is the personal use of self in a positive way that is the best, most effective motivator. And you are their **main** motivator.

Appendix

Practical Exercises

Exercise One

Let's put some of what you've learned into action. Below is an activity experience with a real need for you, as an activity leader, to improve:

> The Activity Director decides it is a beautiful day and everyone in the facility would love to be outside. She calls each unit at lunch to say that she will be outside in fifteen minutes for a program. Only two participants arrive and they leave within ten minutes, stating "it is too cold," and "it's too bright." The Activity Director doesn't understand why the program failed because it is a beautiful day and everyone would love to be outside!

Your Analysis:

Considerations:

- Did the Activity Director consider the real needs of people she was serving, or did she, perhaps, attempt to meet her own need to be outside?
- Was the amount of notice to other staff sufficient? (It was lunch time and they might also be involved in feeding or transporting.)
- What about the lack of sufficient communication to participants in the program, so, if interested, they could be appropriately dressed for their needs (e.g., sweater, hat)?
- What were people expected to do when they got outside? Were chairs set up as needed? Was a program planned with a direction or purpose?
- What other considerations did you think of?

Exercise Two

Write about a recent activity experience you conducted or in which you participated:

Analysis:

Comments:

Did you find ways to improve your own activity or the example of the one you participated in? If so, you are human and open to growth. Realize that motivating others is a precarious skill. And it takes time. The atmosphere could seem "perfect" and still the activity might fail if everyone stays within himself or herself.

On the other hand, the motivation might be there, but the activity failed because the atmosphere is not conducive: e.g., incorrect time of day, group too large or too small, too much distraction, too hot or cold, too few assistants, too much time or too little.

The important thing to know is that your skills and ability to look at the whole activity experience can be improved. What is the secret? It's you and your sincere desire to improve next time and each time you interact with others or plan and conduct an activity. Good luck! And have fun!

References and Additional Reading

Bromley, D. B. (1990). *Behavioral gerontology: Control issues in the psychiatry of aging.* New York, NY: John Wiley & Sons.

Cummings, E. M., Greene, A. L., and Karraker, K. H. (Eds.). (1991). *Life-span developmental psychology: Perspectives on stress and coping.* Hillsdale, NJ: Lawrence Erlbaum Associates.

Erikson, J. (1976). *Activity, recovery, growth: The communal role of planned activities.* New York. NY: W.W. Norton.

Feather, N. T. (Ed.). (1982). *Expectations and actions: Expectancy-value models in psychology.* Hillsdale, NJ: Lawrence Erlbaum Associates.

Frye, V., and Peters, M. (1972). *Therapeutic recreation: It's theory, philosophy, and practice.* Harrisburg, PA: Stackpole Books.

Iso-Ahola, S. E. (1980). *The social psychology of leisure and recreation.* Dubuque, IA: William C. Brown Co.

Lindbergh, A. M. (1975). *Gift from the sea.* New York, NY: Pantheon Books.

Martin, S., and Smith, R. W. (1993) OBRA legislation and recreational activities: Enhancing personal control in nursing homes. *Activities, Adaptation & Aging, 17*(3) 1-14.

Miller, W. R., and Rollnick, S. (1991). *Motivational interviewing.* New York, NY: Guilford Press.

Prochaska, J. O., and DiClemente, C. C. (1982). Transtheoretical therapy: Toward a more integrative model of change. *Psychotherapy: Therapy, Research, and Practice, 19,* 276-288.

Rogers, C. R. (1961). *On becoming a person.* Boston, MA: Houghton Mifflin Co.

Smith, C. P. (1992). *Motivation and personality: Handbook of thematic content analysis.* New York, NY: Cambridge University Press.

Toates, F. (1986). *Motivational systems.* New York, NY: Cambridge University Press.

Witt, P. A., and Ellis, G. (1989). *The Leisure diagnostic battery: Users manual and sample forms.* State College, PA: Venture Publishing, Inc.

Other Books from Venture Publishing

The A•B•Cs of Behavior Change: Skills for Working with Behavior Problems in Nursing Homes
    by Margaret D. Cohn, Michael A. Smyer and Ann L. Horgas
Activity Experiences and Programming Within Long-Term Care
    by Ted Tedrick and Elaine R. Green
The Activity Gourmet
    by Peggy Powers
Advanced Concepts for Geriatric Nursing Assistants
    by Carolyn A. McDonald
Adventure Education
    edited by John C. Miles and Simon Priest
Assessment: The Cornerstone of Activity Programs
    by Ruth Perschbacher
At-Risk Youth and Gangs—A Resource Manual for the Parks and Recreation Professional—Expanded and Updated
    by The California Park and Recreation Society
Behavior Modification in Therapeutic Recreation: An Introductory Learning Manual
    by John Dattilo and William D. Murphy
Benefits of Leisure
    edited by B. L. Driver, Perry J. Brown and George L. Peterson
Benefits of Recreation Research Update
    by Judy M. Sefton and W. Kerry Mummery
Beyond Bingo: Innovative Programs for the New Senior
    by Sal Arrigo, Jr., Ann Lewis and Hank Mattimore

Other Books from Venture Publishing

Both Gains and Gaps: Feminist Perspectives on Women's Leisure
    by Karla Henderson, M. Deborah Bialeschki, Susan M. Shaw and Valeria J. Freysinger

The Community Tourism Industry Imperative—The Necessity, The Opportunities, Its Potential
    by Uel Blank

Dimensions of Choice: A Qualitative Approach to Recreation, Parks, and Leisure Research
    by Karla A. Henderson

Evaluating Leisure Services: Making Enlightened Decisions
    by Karla A. Henderson with M. Deborah Bialeschki

Evaluation of Therapeutic Recreation Through Quality Assurance
    edited by Bob Riley

The Evolution of Leisure: Historical and Philosophical Perspectives
    by Thomas Goodale and Geoffrey Godbey

The Game Finder—A Leader's Guide to Great Activities
    by Annette C. Moore

Great Special Events and Activities
    by Annie Morton, Angie Prosser and Sue Spangler

Inclusive Leisure Services: Responding to the Rights of People with Disabilities
    by John Dattilo

Internships in Recreation and Leisure Services: A Practical Guide for Students
    by Edward E. Seagle, Jr., Ralph W. Smith and Lola M. Dalton

Interpretation of Cultural and Natural Resources
    by Douglas M. Knudson, Ted T. Cable and Larry Beck

Introduction to Leisure Services—7th Edition
    by H. Douglas Sessoms and Karla A. Henderson

Leadership and Administration of Outdoor Pursuits, Second Edition
    by Phyllis Ford and James Blanchard

Leisure And Family Fun (LAFF)
    by Mary Atteberry-Rogers

The Leisure Diagnostic Battery: Users Manual and Sample Forms
    by Peter A. Witt and Gary Ellis

Leisure Diagnostic Battery Computer Software
    by Gary Ellis and Peter A. Witt

Leisure Education: A Manual of Activities and Resources
    by Norma J. Stumbo and Steven R. Thompson

Leisure Education II: More Activities and Resources
    by Norma J. Stumbo

Leisure Education Program Planning: A Systematic Approach
    by John Dattilo and William D. Murphy

Leisure in Your Life: An Exploration, Fourth Edition
    by Geoffrey Godbey
A Leisure of One's Own: A Feminist Perspective on Women's Leisure
    by Karla Henderson, M. Deborah Bialeschki, Susan M. Shaw and
    Valeria J. Freysinger
Leisure Services in Canada: An Introduction
    by Mark S. Searle and Russell E. Brayley
Leveraging the Benefits of Parks and Recreation: The Phoenix Project
    by The California Park and Recreation Society
Marketing for Parks, Recreation, and Leisure
    by Ellen L. O'Sullivan
Models of Change in Municipal Parks and Recreation: A Book of Innovative Case Studies
    edited by Mark E. Havitz
Outdoor Recreation Management: Theory and Application, Third Edition
    by Alan Jubenville and Ben Twight
Planning Parks for People
    by John Hultsman, Richard L. Cottrell and Wendy Zales Hultsman
The Process of Recreation Programming Theory and Technique, Third Edition
    by Patricia Farrell and Herberta M. Lundegren
Protocols for Recreation Therapy Programs
    edited by Jill Kelland, along with the Recreation Therapy Staff at
    Alberta Hospital Edmonton
Quality Management: Applications for Therapeutic Recreation
    edited by Bob Riley
Recreation and Leisure: Issues in an Era of Change, Third Edition
    edited by Thomas Goodale and Peter A. Witt
The Recreation Connection to Self-Esteem—A Resource Manual for the Park, Recreation and Community Services Professional
    by The California Park and Recreation Society
Recreation Programming and Activities for Older Adults
    by Jerold E. Elliott and Judith A. Sorg-Elliott
Reference Manual for Writing Rehabilitation Therapy Treatment Plans
    by Penny Hogberg and Mary Johnson
Research in Therapeutic Recreation: Concepts and Methods
    edited by Marjorie J. Malkin and Christine Z. Howe
A Social History of Leisure Since 1600
    by Gary Cross
The Sociology of Leisure
    by John R. Kelly and Geoffrey Godbey

A Study Guide for National Certification in Therapeutic Recreation
    by Gerald O'Morrow and Ron Reynolds
Therapeutic Recreation: Cases and Exercises
    by Barbara C. Wilhite and M. Jean Keller
Therapeutic Recreation in the Nursing Home
    by Linda Buettner and Shelley L. Martin
Therapeutic Recreation Protocol for Treatment of Substance Addictions
    by Rozanne W. Faulkner
A Training Manual for Americans With Disabilities Act Compliance in Parks and Recreation Settings
    by Carol Stensrud
Understanding Leisure and Recreation: Mapping the Past, Charting the Future
    edited by Edgar L. Jackson and Thomas L. Burton

 Venture Publishing, Inc.
1999 Cato Avenue
State College, PA 16801

Phone: (814) 234-4561; FAX: (814) 234-1651